Seasonal Fires

Seasonal Fires

new and selected poems

INGRID DE KOK

Seven Stories Press

NEW YORK ✦ TORONTO ✦ LONDON ✦ MELBOURNE

Seven Stories Press
140 Watts Street
New York, NY 10013
http://www.sevenstories.com/

In Canada: Publishers Group Canada, 250A Carlton Street, Toronto, ON M5A 2L1

In the UK: Turnaround Publisher Services Ltd., Unit 3, Olympia Trading Estate,
Coburg Road, Wood Green, London N22 6TZ

In Australia: Palgrave Macmillan, 627 Chapel Street, South Yarra, VIC 3141

College professors may order examination copies of Seven Stories Press titles for a
free six-month trial period. To order, visit www.sevenstories.com/textbook/
or send a fax on school letterhead to 212.226.1411.

Book design by Phoebe Hwang

LIBRARY OF CONGRESS CATALOGING-IN-PUBLICATION DATA
De Kok, Ingrid, 1951–
Seasonal fires : new and selected poems / Ingrid de Kok.
— 1st Seven Stories Press ed.
p. cm.
ISBN-13: 978-1-58322-718-3 (pbk. : alk. paper)
ISBN-10: 1-58322-718-0 (pbk. : alk. paper)
I. Title.
PR9369.3.C36S43 2006
821'.914—dc22
2005035935

Printed in the USA

9 8 7 6 5 4 3 2 1

For Luke Fiske

Acknowledgments

Some of the new poems in this collection first appeared (some in slightly different versions) in the following journals and books: *Carapace; New Contrast; Freedom Spring: Ten Years On; Johannesburg Circa Now: Photography and the City; Imagination in a Troubled Space: A South African Reader; Curiosity* CLXXV: *A Paper Cabinet; Capilano Review;* and *Poetry International.*

I would like to thank the Civitella Ranieri Foundation for a 2004 fellowship at the Center in Umbria, during which some of the new poems were completed. Thanks, too, to Karen Press, Gus Ferguson, Jenny Penberthy, and Tony Morphet for assistance in the preparation of this book.

Contents

POEMS FROM *FAMILIAR GROUND* (1988)

15   To drink its water
17   Sun, aloe, rain
19   Our Sharpeville
21   At this resort
23   My father would not show us
25   Shadows behind, before
27   Two places, two dreams
28   Ruth in the corn
29   The two Sherpas
30   Woman, leaning away
32   Dolphin eater
33   Enduring your devil
34   Woman in the glass
36   To a would-be lover
38   Words of love
40   Visitor
41   Arrangement: a poem for myself
43   This thing we learn from others

45 On her way home
47 Road through Lesotho
48 Stones, sky, radio
49 *Al wat kind is*
51 Small passing

POEMS FROM *TRANSFER* (1997)

57 Transfer
59 Keeper
61 Ground wave
62 Still life
63 What everyone should know about grief
65 In the Cappuchin ossuarium, Rome
67 Cape Town morning
68 Cape Town by day
69 Cape Town by night
70 At the commission
71 The resurrection bush
72 Mending
73 My mother's house hold
75 Young boy juggling
77 After forty
78 Safe delivery
79 Wattle-eyes
80 Text of necessity
81 Night space
82 Inner note
84 Brush stroke
85 Aubade
86 Stay here

POEMS FROM *TERRESTRIAL THINGS* (2002)

89 Spring custom

92 Birds at Bellagio

93 Lizards at San Michele

94 Merchants in Venice

96 Parts of speech

97 The Archbishop chairs the first session

99 How to mourn in a room full of questions

100 Tongue-tied

101 What kind of man?

105 Revenge of the imagination

107 A commander grieves on his own

109 The transcriber speaks

110 The sound engineer

112 Some there be

113 Body parts

114 Sticks on stone

116 A few questions

117 Frightened of the dark

119 In the cage

120 Sirens sounding

121 William Kamanga

123 My father's books

125 A death foretold

126 In a northern city, suddenly

128 Into the sun

130 The head of the household

132 Women and children first

133 The child at the lights

134 Compassionate leave

NEW POEMS

BODY MAPS

139 Reparation
140 Too long a sacrifice
142 Bring the statues back
144 In times of war
146 Pilgrimage
148 Treasury
151 "The Fear of God is the Beginning of Knowledge"
152 Body maps
155 Threnody
156 Wishing in moonlight
158 Child stretching
160 Letter from childhood
162 When children leave
163 Will
164 Notes for that week
168 Death arrives
170 Death notices
172 Time to go
173 The eclipse of the sun
175 Kalahari campsite

SKETCHES FROM A SUMMER NOTEBOOK

179 Letter home
181 Umbrian shutters
182 Walking back late at night
183 Solitaire at Fronzola
184 La Traviata
185 Sunflowers
186 In the chimney

Poems from
Familiar Ground

(1988)

TO DRINK ITS WATER

1

Home is where the heart is:
a tin can tied to a stray dog.

The only truth is home truth:
preserves on the winter shelf.

Those who carry their homes on their backs
live for hundreds of years,
moving inch by inch from birth to lagoon.

2

Beside the beaten path
to the veld where I once played,
dry riverbed and unwashed clothes
grey lizards on the rocks.
My shadow squats in the shade of a thorn
where children sift and store
the remnants of corroded bins.
Over the path, the rocks, the tree,
marauding sky, fiercer than memory.

3

In a hot country
light is a leper,
water the eye of a goat
on the fork of an honoured guest.

The tap in the camp drips onto the bone of the gum.

And those in the cool green houses,
owners of the sweet white water,
owners of the bins and wells,
die swollen, host and guest of a herd of eyes
washing within them.

4

To return home, you have to drink its water,
in a drought you have to drink its water,
even from the courtyard well,
the water blossoming in the gut,
or brackish, from a burning trough,
flypaper on your tongue,
pooling your hands,
bending when you drink.

5

Home is where the heart is:
husk of heat on the back.

The sky enters into the skin,
the sky's red ants
crawl over the shoulders.

This bending body is my only body.
I bend and drink
the shadow in the water.

SUN, ALOE, RAIN

I

On the edge of scrub, where I grew up,
there were many veld fires in the brittle summer
and the heat in the heat consumed itself
and the air and land grew blacker and blacker.

I once saw a fire move like
coral lightning across the sand
after a meercat maddened
by the cremating arc.

And once, when the heat was like sandpaper, like scorpions,
I saw a salt pan under the high hard sun,
and watched the flamingoes rise, startled,
their underwings protected and pink.

In the veld were thorn trees in patches
like the dregs of other, imaginary gardens,
except in spring, when sticky with yellow life
they had another name, mimosa.

And in the gardens there were always aloes, sharp as blood,
and leathery cannas, all male flowers.
No one has yet put aloes and cannas
into a sweet-smelling basket or pitcher of water.

2

I remember going to a party,
seven and very severe,
in my sober dress two inches over the knee
and my high forehead and my mother's way.
There were lots of children
hiding and seeking, in shifting alliance,
while on the verandah the dog panted
and hopscotch lines simmered on the driveway.
I sat, more sullen than shy, licking my icecream carefully,
hating the aloes and cannas in their tended rows.

Playing games, no one noticed
the air was swelling, heavy on our heads,
and the ground sour with expectation.

Then the storm broke, an exploding rock,
a detonating jewel, its pieces of hot hail
knocking the cannas flat into the earth, puncturing aloes,
and the rain leapt over and over us.

When it was time to go, I ran
across the muddy grass, my back to an imagined breeze,
the yellow ribbons in my hair, loose and lovely,
breaking like waves against my long, thin neck.

OUR SHARPEVILLE

I was playing hopscotch on the slate
when miners roared past in lorries,
their arms raised, signals at a crossing,
their chanting foreign and familiar,
like the call and answer of road gangs
across the veld, building hot arteries
from the heart of the Transvaal mine.

I ran to the gate to watch them pass.
And it seemed like a great caravan
moving across the desert to an oasis
I remembered from my Sunday School book:
olive trees, a deep jade pool,
men resting in clusters after a long journey,
the danger of the mission still around them,
and night falling, its silver stars just like the ones
you got for remembering your Bible texts.

Then my grandmother called from behind the front door,
her voice a stiff broom over the steps:
"Come inside; they do things to little girls."

For it was noon, and there was no jade pool.
Instead, a pool of blood that already had a living name
and grew like a shadow as the day lengthened.
The dead, buried in voices that reached even my gate,
the chanting men on the ambushed trucks,
these were not heroes in my town,
but maulers of children,
doing things that had to remain nameless.
And our Sharpeville was this fearful thing
that might tempt us across the wellswept streets.

If I had turned I would have seen
brocade curtains drawn tightly across sheer net ones,
known there were eyes behind both,
heard the dogs pacing in the locked yard next door.
But, walking backwards, all I felt was shame,
at being a girl, at having been found at the gate,
at having heard my grandmother lie
and at my fear her lie might be true.
Walking backwards, called back,
I returned to the closed rooms, home.

AT THIS RESORT

Tropical plants fringe the sea,
voluptuous branches, heavy with steam and heat
rot onto the moving dunes.
In front of the verandah here
berries swell, red,
crack open like eggs,
their seeds glow poison,
irradiate, glow red.
But for all we know they might have healing properties,
nourish birds, oil flaccid feathers:
they might have saved us.

Really, there is no secret in the view.
I put it there.
No loss at all but landscape, landscape.
The tree bears nothing
that cannot be identified.
The rule of thumb is:
do not eat what even birds avoid.
But here we cannot tell which are the birds.

At the edge of the resort,
beyond the shop, dining room,
bowling greens, the children's trampoline,
the stars dip their wicks
into the waxen fever trees
and shadowy men and boys throat
across the low lagoon.

So lose again a father, lover, son,
to the dark sand
that no one cares to tread upon
unless it is the only pathway
to the rocks and then the hills.

And all along the broken water,
women wardens stand
shaking hands forever at the church door,
greeting the mourners with their dark lapels,
while the coffins heave themselves into the sea.

MY FATHER WOULD NOT SHOW US

Which way do we face to talk to the dead?
—Rainer Maria Rilke

❦

My father's face
five days dead
is organized for me to see.

It's cold in here
and the borrowed coffin gleams unnaturally;
the pine one has not yet been delivered.

Half-expected this inverted face
but not the soft, for some reason
unfrozen collar of his striped pyjamas.

This is the last time I am allowed
to remember my childhood as it might have been:
a louder, braver place,
crowded, a house with a tin roof
being hailed upon, and voices rising,
my father's wry smile, his half-turned face.

My father would not show us how to die.
He hid, he hid away.
Behind the curtains where his life had been,
the florist's flowers curling into spring,
he lay inside, he lay.

He could recall the rag-and-bone man
passing his mother's gate in the morning light.
Now the tunnelling sound of the dogs next door;
everything he hears is white.

My father could not show us how to die.
He turned, he turned away.
Under the counterpane, without one call
or word or name,
face to the wall, he lay.

SHADOWS BEHIND, BEFORE

Sky, almond and chalk,
fields bleached with old use,
the highway a silver arrow
through the heart of it all.
If I keep travelling this way
will I know when I've reached the site,
knowledge trickling through my fingers
my hands so full of its soil?

There are two myths of possession here:
the myth of the exile, wanderer,
carrying loss like a bomb under his coat,
a load of winter wood on his back,
mercenary of his own heart's plunder;
and the myth of the householder,
partisan of familiar fields,
who builds his past from mud and water
and his future with the same.

No matter if he visits a valley, the exile
watches from a copse on a windless hill.
But a native in his own place cannot afford
to speculate on the distance to his father's barn.
Each in silence walks a pathway
to a pond that barely moves,
but one turns his back on his own long shadow
and one watches his shadow lead him deep into winter.

In this chill evening ride
the houses buckle into the road's long belt.
Behind a window a woman watches me pass,
matching my eyes as they snatch and drop her.
She sees me, promised unknown distance,
free or urgent to be travelling away;
I see her draw water from a deep metallic well,
I see her candles for the dead.

TWO PLACES, TWO DREAMS

My child, brought from his own country,
is sleeping in a Cape bed
where the black south-easter
delivers boats and fish
to his hot summer dream
of kelp and tentacles
that hang like fingers from his hands.

In his other dream
pines, like ravens blue with cold,
fly into the ice,
and snow falling from low branches
sifts onto his thin chest.

As he calls in the dark,
"Come," "Go,"
the sea invades the low lagoon
and the red cardinal shaken from his sheet
flies into its dense natal tree.

RUTH IN THE CORN

Ontario, 1984

The geese overhead,
the autumn hieroglyph
that everyone can read
and understand.

When you who live and know this place,
when you watch them pass,
you remember their return
even as you lose the sound
of their high migration.

But the others, who see
plantations of olives,
the Southern Cross,
the scrub on the edge of the desert
in the pattern of flight,
when they follow the long geese
overhead, leaving forever,
they want to sing of the south,
even of the southern cities,
even of the small hot rooms.

Sick for home are those watching people
when the fall sky moves its migrating birds.

THE TWO SHERPAS

Today, Canadian mountain climber Laurie Skreslet reached the summit
of Mount Everest. With him were two Sherpas.
—Report by the Canadian Broadcasting Corporation
on The National News

Donkeys, clearly, special mountain ones,
or computers to connect The Mountain
with The National.
Or lungs, or esoteric climbing gear,
one for each foot.

Or let's just call them Dan and Sam Sherpa.
Dan didn't need oxygen until the last 200 feet.
Sam had been there twice before.
They might even be good in a crisis,
might even know the way.

Every Canadian deserves one of those Sherpas.
I want one for myself, whatever it is.

WOMAN, LEANING AWAY

He hands it to me
as if it were her wedding ring
the picture of his mother
remoter than the island
she couldn't leave.

She is leaning away from herself,
from the photograph, from us,
towards something out there,
a tree or stone or colour.
Her dress is soft, unstylish,
and perhaps her hands are folded.
He will give her anything,
corals, pearls, all his photographs of her
if she will turn just once
to see him watching her
the way one watches for a bird
whose sound in the dense green
promises shape just before it is silent again.

I think of her as a woman
whose eyes must have been grey
who said nothing of her own mother
or the things she heard as a child
on a balcony over the narrow streets
leaning towards the sea.

When her children left for the mainland
she may have laid out her clothes on the bed,
opened the shutters to air the empty rooms,
then turned to stand,
stiller than the photograph,
near a trellis of sweet smells
so thick it concealed the hills.

Only afterwards
lying beside him in the cool
I realize this was a test
to see if I too would lean
away from him and the open window
while I looked on the photograph
of his silent mother.

DOLPHIN EATER

There was nothing else to eat.
So I ate the dolphin
and asked my friend
never ever to tell.

Like lightning
that night
sea struck me
and I screamed in my sleep
for a boat to take me back
to the first shore
where I had eaten no dolphin.

In my eyes dolphins dancing
in the bay close to shore
a gift of the evening tide
to the strollers on the beach.
In my mouth, dolphin.

I tricked the silent ferryman,
gave beads for land,
and the silver cargo of the dhow
discharged into my palm.

Nothing will save me now
in the waves off the cliffs.
I will not be brought home
on the leeside of a dolphin's fin.

ENDURING YOUR DEVIL

In the cottage the candles flickered for sanity.
You say you were alone except for
wind off the cliffs and the devil.

You could not shut the door
that swung wide into that place.
Even the crucifix could not do that.

You ask me to remember
the blasted heath, the slouching beast,
the Florence of Savanarola.

But I hear only your thin words:
"I stayed awake all night
watching the open door, keeping the evil out."

It's no use looking for comfort in the Apocrypha,
in the images you subpoena
at the crossroads where suicides are buried.

You cannot survive this devil
with an arsenal of texts and spells.
You cannot keep him out with a guard at the gate.

Blow out the candles,
Let the cliff winds blow.
Poor windswept devil, take him in,
Get to know him well.

WOMAN IN THE GLASS

I am not the woman in the train
who pulls your hand between her legs
and then looks out of the window.

I am not the woman with the henna hair
in a city street, who never says a word
but beckons you, beckons you.

Nor am I the woman in the glass
who looks at you look at her
and the glass smokes over.

Nor the woman who holds you
whilst you call out the names of lost lovers
as you will call out this one.

Nor am I the woman in the dark
whose silence is the meteor
in the sky of your conversation.

That woman:
bent over, offering her sex to you
like a globe of garlic, asking for nothing;
the one without fingerprints,
hiding in the amulet of your protection;
the one surrounded by photographers
printing her supple smile, her skin:
that woman.

I stand to the side and watch her,
widow-virgin, burn on your pyre.
Acrobat falling into a net of ash,
in the flames her mouth drips wax,
her eyebrows peel off,
her sex unstitches its tiny mirrors.

Your woman: cousin, sister, twin.
You want her burning, distant, dumb.
I want to save, and tear, her tongue.

TO A WOULD-BE LOVER

I once knew a man who made love
with pockets of iron filings.
The machines were oiled, the pistons shone,
we were stapled together and sent through a shute.

And you would probably balance
like a gymnast on the cross-bar,
just before the triple turn,
with the air still, audience still,
energy parallel with intention.

I cannot love athletes or makers of metal things
or anyone associated with Concorde.
I like the sillier body, earthbound,
with its many joints and dents:
a squat figure on a sweaty mat.
The delicious fiction, love,
must dangle its infinitives,
forget to close its clauses,
offer alternative endings,
a hero whose shirt hangs out
and a heroine who trips over the bed
because her contacts are lost under the sink.

Praise be the inelegance of ordinary love
when the children on the street
are skidding on skateboards
and the doorbell rings and has to be ignored
when the pillows are too soft
and the feet are much too cold.

So, pyrotechnic suitor,
your skin is far too sleek,
your arms too architectural,
your timing much too neat.
I'm sure you'll find another
to watch you in the mirror
but I must refuse your offer
and decline to conjugate.

WORDS OF LOVE

1

He said:
"Are you happy?"
"Are you alright?"
"What are you thinking?"
"Are you alright?"
He said: "These words,
the fetishes of early anxious love."

She said:
"How strange and how familiar
the breathing of a new lover."
"Are you alright?"
"Are you still there?"
She said: "The mist at this time of year
confuses everything."

2

Oh how we swallow, how then we carry
in our pouches the words of our lovers
as if they are our own.
Our mouths are icing tubes and vases
and we lipstick the words of love
onto hall mirrors, onto ourselves,
or have them implanted
silicon deep in our pointed breasts.

Knowing the thoughts of the beloved,
having the same thoughts,
or something close enough, like false teeth,
caps, crowns, bridges,
letting them rise out of our mouths
into bubbles, into an adult comic strip:
this is called *love*.

Till the bubbles blow off the page,
are spiked on thorntrees,
collapse like Chinese lanterns,
or we chew them like gum,
the words of our lovers,
gag, spit out at last
a trickle of sounds
more like our own:
this is called *betrayal*.

3

No woman ever says
"It's in the pipeline"
even in countries with large oil reserves
and women on the rigs.

VISITOR

When you turn to me, carrying your weight on your side
like a gypsy with a pail, I must stroke you cleverly,
gently, taking care to be silent: sounds carry.

You are a guest here, and your pain is unfamiliar to me
even when you turn like this into my hospitable hands
and I have to call you my own.

On a still afternoon, you visit your request on me
that I cannot answer, cannot refuse.
You are thinner than I remember.

ARRANGEMENT: A POEM FOR MYSELF

In the room with a round mahogany table
I recognize myself, arranging the flowers.
From spring somewhere else I bring
freesias, anemone, yellow roses
and jasmine, fragrant as water.
There is only one rule:
from all sides the arrangement must look perfect.
It must not prefer the window seat
or the large oil painting
or even myself, who appears to be judging.

But freesias are so light
they want to fly like butterflies above the other flowers.
I let them rise and settle
while the roses drink and drink,
water entering them like blood.
One jasmine blossom is so Japanese
it belongs in a vase by itself
in another room, with mirrors.
Stems must be cut to size.
Anything brown has to go.
Even one shooting star
that scatters its petals like ore
on the round mahogany table
must be gathered into newspaper
and carried from the room.

This culling of flowers like young impala
they say is "for the sake of the whole,"
but what I mean is that
I have to choose flowers
that will live in this vase
as if it is the earth
and the death of flowers
that cannot transform themselves,
even when my hands are full of their sacrifice,
is like air in my lungs.

THIS THING WE LEARN FROM OTHERS

From the hitchhiker whose head
falls against your shoulder in his sleep
as you swerve in the dark rain,
from two small boys waving
at a Safari Tours bus,
from others, that stowaway for instance,
who gave himself up because
from his hiding place
he couldn't smell the sea,
and from people who bury their dogs
in gardens, at night,
remembering the date until they are old.

They say if your mother held you
on her right side, head in the moist curve
of her arm, you are lonely,
and if she held you on her left,
her breast breathing into your ear,
you are lonely.

To be thus
is what we should have expected.

Only, at spring tide,
its moon just a glance
over the wet uncovered miles of sand,
the rocks white and black mica in the dark,
and waves which had buried themselves
at our feet, now trebling quietly
far out there
made us come close
to the fire on the beach,
made us think it possible
to stay that way,
scooping warm coals into the heart.

ON HER WAY HOME

For Mary Anne

This is her favourite view on her way home:
when the road leans suddenly
towards a grey outcrop of rock and shadow,
a hill pockmarked by aloes,
when the sky is dead clear, the sun dead centre,
and the others driving past
turn to their conversations
about resorts along the river further on.

She stopped once to walk in the place.
Her children ran ahead, looking for snakes,
feeling the heat fill their shoes
like thick dust, imagining leopards and vultures
and the weapons they would use to subdue them.
The sun settled, a horsefly on her head:
she would not brush it away.

Far away on a black flank she saw the children,
grey goats on another continent,
heard from over the hill the stuck sound
of cars immobile in liquefied tar,
bent to see the order of large red ants on the sand,
felt their filings on her bare legs.

Heat bearing down
on her neck, behind her knees.
In her head sun stroking her,
clay beads of sweat in her head,
in her pupils blacker and blacker.
The skull of a sheep made her think
of erecting gazebos in the place
and she laughed out loud
so far from the river
remembering the futile shade of willows.

When the boys came upon her
looking straight into the sun,
they were large white rings in her viewing.
Their hands burning, they dozed fitfully
the half hour home, not noticing
how she stopped singing
when the road entered their valley
shining with the ribbons of irrigated colour.

ROAD THROUGH LESOTHO

From over the corrugated hills we are sighted
driving along the inhospitable road, casting a lumpy shadow.
His arms flapping, mouth shuttering,
the boy who cares for his father's cattle
hurdles towards us, a missile of expectations.

We keep on moving. Will he reach us before we swerve
beyond, into a village of women and children?
The clouds muscle. Thunder and electric light.
No time to stop, play Lady Bountiful.

But there he is before us, blocking escape,
a toll gate into Africa.
His breath grinds dry and hard.
He has three clay oxen for sale.
"Ten cents missus, ten cents missus?"

Am I a Ten Cents Missus? I do not know his name.
He bends his knees of warring bones.
His hands are curved and small.
I am a visitor with things in my pockets.
It is shameful to give trifles to children.

But unsmilingly he claims his payment,
not caring for my guidebook scruples.
Herder of cattle, other plans in his head,
he has been on the hills all day, waiting for us.

STONES, SKY, RADIO

Around the roots of the tree
the children are dicing with stones.
The sky is immense as the sky,
the sun is as hot as the noonday sun,
the red ants are industrious as ants.
The children are dicing with stones.

Across the grey veld a man is walking.
He is neither young nor old.
He is holding a stick and kicking a tin
and walks like a man walking
across the veld in the dust.

In the distance a radio crackles
out of a cluster of huts.
This is not a sign of life.
It is a radio in a village.

There is nothing else to see or hear
at this time and place, apparently.
The children are still dicing with stones.

AL WAT KIND IS

They took all that was child in the house.
—Resident of Victoria West in the Cape, reporting on
police action in the town.

They took all that was child
and in the dark closed room
visions of a ripe split melon
were at the tip of a knife
they held to the child's dry tongue.

All that was child
lies on the tarmac;
the intestines spill
like beans from a sack,
seaweed from the winter sea.

The bird of state has talons
and shit that drops like lead.
Its metal wings corrode the streets,
it hatches pools of blood.

A stone against a tank is a stone against a tank
but a bullet in a child's chest rips into the heart of the house.

But when in time the single stones
compact their weight and speed together,
roll up the incline towards the lamvanger's lair,
crushing sand into rock, rock into boulder,
boulder into mountain, mountain into sky,
then the lungs of the bird will choke,
the wings will blister and crack,
at last the eyes will glaze, defeated.

And this torn light,
this long torn light
will repair itself
out of the filaments of children,
and all that is child will return to the house,
will open the doors of the house.

SMALL PASSING

*For a woman whose baby died stillborn, and who was told by a man
to stop mourning, "because the trials and horrors suffered daily
by black women in this country are more significant
than the loss of one white child."*

I

In this country you may not
suffer the death of your stillborn,
remember the last push into shadow and silence,
the useless wires and cords on your stomach,
the nurse's face, the walls, the afterbirth in a basin.
Do not touch your breasts
still full of purpose.
Do not circle the house,
pack, unpack the small clothes.
Do not lie awake at night hearing
the doctor say "It was just as well"
and "You can have another."
In this country you may not
mourn small passings.

See: the newspaper boy in the rain
will sleep tonight in a doorway.
The woman in the busline
may next month be on a train
to a place not her own.
The baby in the backyard now
will be sent to a tired aunt,
grow chubby, then lean,
return a stranger.
Mandela's daughter tried to find her father
through the glass. She thought they'd let her touch him.

And this woman's hands are so heavy when she dusts
the photographs of other children
they fall to the floor and break.
Clumsy woman, she moves so slowly
as if in a funeral rite.

On the pavements the nannies meet.
These are legal gatherings.
They talk about everything, about home,
while the children play among them,
their skins like litmus, their bonnets clean.

2

Small wrist in the grave.
Baby no one carried live
between houses, among trees.
Child shot running,
stones in his pocket,
boy's swollen stomach
full of hungry air.
Girls carrying babies
not much smaller than themselves.
Erosion. Soil washed down to the sea.

3

I think these mothers dream
headstones of the unborn.
Their mourning rises like a wall
no vine will cling to.
They will not tell you your suffering is white.
They will not say it is just as well.
They will not compete for the ashes of infants.
I think they may say to you:
Come with us to the place of mothers.
We will stroke your flat empty belly,
let you weep with us in the dark,
and arm you with one of our babies
to carry home on your back.

Poems from
Transfer

(1997)

TRANSFER

All the family dogs are dead.
A borrowed one, its displaced hip
at an angle to its purebred head,
bays at a siren's emergency climb
whining from the motorway.
Seven strangers now have keys
to the padlock on the gate,
where, instead of lights, a mimosa tree
burns its golden blurred bee-fur
to lead you to the door.

"So many leaves, too many trees"
says the gardener who weekly
salvages an ordered edge;
raking round the rusted rotary hoe
left standing where my uncle last
cranked it hard to clear a space
between the trees, peach orchard,
nectarine and plum, to prove
that he at least could move
the future's rankness to another place.

Forty years ago the house was built
to hold private unhappiness intact,
safe against mobile molecular growths
of city, developers and blacks.
Now rhubarb spurs grow wild and sour;
the mulberries, the ducks and bantams gone.
In the fishpond's sage-green soup
its fraying goldfish decompose the sun,
wax-white lilies float upon the rot.
And leaves in random piles are burning.

Townhouses circle the inheritance.
The fire station and franchised inn
keep neighbourhood watch over its fate.
The municipality leers over the gate,
complains of dispossession and neglect,
dark tenants and the broken fence.
But all the highveld birds are here,
weighing their metronomic blossoms
upon the branches in the winter air.
And the exiles are returning.

KEEPER

The riverine forest
once stored its light
beneath damp canopies of trees,
where vines knotted bright berries
and flycatchers hawked
in the heat's filigree.

Now above the banks
of the dried Luvuvhu river,
carcasses bleach black,
fevered baboons quiver,
and the keeper of Pafuri,
drought's carapace,
asks us for razorblades,
sugar, lard, toothpaste,
stamps and news of camp
as he tends the picnic place.

In rigid sunlight
he sweeps the sand
repolishes the tap
riddles the ashes and recounts:
"The rain has gone.
The river has gone.
God has gone.
The lions keep me awake at night."

Then he shuffles past our car
to his bamboo shack
and remembered birdsong,
summer storms, fresh animal tracks.

GROUND WAVE

Just below the cottage door
our moraine stairway of lemon trees,
strelitzia quills and oleander shrub
steps to the sea and deeper terraces.
The warming wind, concertina on the slope,
coaxes open the bulbul's throat,
the figtree's testicular green globes
and camellia's white evening flux.

Behind the house we feel
the mountain's friction against our backs.
Deep fissures are predicted by the almanac,
earth and trees heaving to the shore.
Scorpions come in at night
for cool killings on the flagstone floor.

STILL LIFE

The woman is wild.
The child has grown
away from this place
to a view of its own.

The woman is still.
The child has gone
behind the hill
foreign moons shine on.

The woman's alive.
The child was led
from summer ground.
The child is fled.

The woman yields the cavity,
renounces daily care,
grants the earth its gravity,
the sky its horizontal stare.

WHAT EVERYONE SHOULD KNOW
ABOUT GRIEF

"What everyone should know about grief"
is why I buy the magazine.
Between aerobic virtue on one page
and the thrills of Machu Picchu on another
grief finds its marketable stage.

The living tell their chronicles
of hurt and lost and dead.
In syncopated copy they rehearse
"the cost of rage," "the comfort of belief,"
in words and captioned movements of the head.

The story proffers help:
advises talking as the healing cure,
commends long walks, and therapies,
assures the grieving that they will endure,
and then it gently cautions: let go, move on.

But everyone knows sorrow is incurable:
a bruised and jagged scar
in the rift valley of the body;
shrapnel seeded in the skin;
undoused burning pyres of war.

And grief is one thing nearly personal,
a hairline fracture in an individual skull;
homemade elegy which sounds its keening
in the scarred heart's well;
where it is too deep to reach

the ladder of light
sent down from land above,
where hands write words
to work the winch
to plumb the shaft below.

IN THE CAPPUCHIN OSSUARIUM, ROME

I've been to stare here twice before,
led by a silent monk, and shown
shrunken skulls, stooped skeletons,
tarsals, shins and pelvic bones.

This time he points me to a sign
above the scaffoldings of sin
and when I've read the warning text
we share a disinterred tight grin.

This cartilaginous vocation
is what I cannot flee:
"Where you are, we once were.
Where we are, you shall be."

I breathe the dampness of the crypt,
smell sawdust and the acrid horn,
and suck dark death under my flesh
until I'm shriven, rabid,

burning to petrify a wreath,
my gristle for God's glory,
yearning to count my rosary
boned memento mori.

The relics, God's Medusa locks,
fix my eyes, arrest escape.
I turn obedient to the monk
who can't outlive and can't forgive

the light outside, the fragrant air,
loud voices on the fountained streets,
and children on the pathways home,
their bony, bare, small feet.

CAPE TOWN MORNING

Winter has passed. The wind is back.
Window panes rattle old rust,
summer rising.

Street children sleep, shaven mummies in sacks,
eyelids weighted by dreams of coins,
beneath them treasure of small knives.

Flower sellers add fresh blossoms
to yesterday's blooms, sour buckets
filled and spilling.

And trucks digest the city's sediment
men gloved and silent
in the municipal jaws.

CAPE TOWN BY DAY

A marshland of fog and gas
muffles the commerce of sound,
turns Cape Town into Venice

as the light on the dock laps
tackle, cranes, yards, grain elevators,
suspending them in tidal anchorage.

Shimmering like a promise, the yellow mirage
prepares sailors for the city,
its irradiated bowl.

CAPE TOWN BY NIGHT

From Signal Hill
on Valentine's night
car alarms rouse
the last romantics.

City lights
flicker, on, off.

Underneath,
gaunt men in doorways
and ransacked women
key back rooms.

Taxis sidle to their ranks,
newspapers blow.

AT THE COMMISSION

In the retelling
no one remembers
whether he was carrying a grenade
or if his pent up body
exploded on contact with
horrors to come.

Would it matter to know
the detail called truth
since, fast forwarded,
the ending is the same,
over and over?

The questions, however intended,
all lead away from him
alone there, running for his life.

THE RESURRECTION BUSH

The desiccated soil only raises
archaeological relics,
grey shale, stunted bush
and this dead clump of sticks

no one noticed between the rocks
till the ranger broke a stalk
as if to chew or crumble it
while we climbed and talked.

Purgatorial bouquet,
dry brush of drier summer,
then placed in water overnight
drifts in a porous coma.

Just as Egyptian sheaves,
delivered from their vacuum tomb
as dormant seed, air
inspired to corn again,

so in one day stick turns to stalk,
in three, gold nodules nudge and stir,
then tinder flares into tendril fire:
a xerophilous shooting star.

Scorched bushveld stoic,
shriveled, sown in stone,
its sap revived, sprouts green again
in one chance cup of rain.

MENDING

In and out, behind, across.
The formal gesture binds the cloth.
The stitchery's a surgeon's rhyme,
a Chinese stamp, a pantomime

of print. Then spoor. Then trail of red.
Scabs rise, stigmata from the thread.
A cotton chronicle congealed.
A histogram of welts and weals.

The woman plies her ancient art.
Her needle sutures as it darts,
scoring, scripting, scarring, stitching,
the invisible mending of the heart.

MY MOTHER'S HOUSE HOLD

My mother held us to her.
This made friends chafe and sting,
or want her for their own.

There we four were, dragging our feet
backwards and forwards to her love,
trying to keep a secret of ourselves,

while the house filled up with
other people's children.
Perhaps she stole them away.

Now there are more,
those children's children,
an undertow of love.

Watching them, she plays
the same tune I heard at seven:
early anarchic Nat King Cole.

Tender, fatalistic,
ur-mothering,
learnt between the wars.

My mother says its harder
to love a happy person than a sad one.
They need you so much less.

She says she'll put a plastic bag
over her own head
when she wants to die,

not rely on squeamish us
to do the right,
the braver thing.

My mother holds us to her.
This makes friends chafe and sting
and want her for their own.

YOUNG BOY JUGGLING

Legs apart, weighted
by the romance of a trick,
he levitates his cargo,
quick wrist flicking
three sticks clicking
three balls chained by air
tumbling, rising:
ball of the eye,
ball of the palm,
ball of the foot.

He juggles space and gravity
to conjure hazardous rules
out of a sleight of limbs:
the rule of extremity,
where you hold only to let go;
the rule of exposure,
where nothing is held close to the chest;
and the gambler's drill,
which makes devices
look like natural skill.

Travelling exhibit,
fast on his feet,
ego extravaganza
patter, swank, cheat.
In the mirror of his
infatuated trance
quicksilver gypsy
juggles back at him
his career of feinting,
dodging, catching chance.

This is a tableau of display,
(young shaman of the impossible)
before hormones begin to whirl like blackfly
around green's stickiness in spring.

AFTER FORTY

Got half-way with this gene basket,
two birth marks and slasto cellulite.
Hitched a longish ride
with a one of a kind thumbprint,
astigmatic vision and maybe original sin.

Now life's a honeycomb, an anagram,
ammonite, ant trap, knot;
alarm clock set for the same time every morning,
limping iambic footprint, warning trochee cough;
dot-to-dot puzzle on its way to being completed,
meals on wheels, rolling downhill.

So much for the family photograph:
the crisp child posed in front
of her past like a fifties filmstar;
a fledgling imperial eagle
in front of her future.

SAFE DELIVERY

For Jonah Lewis

I claim kin, giddy newborn sprite
since you were conceived after the close dancing
of your begetters and deliverers
in my living room late one August night.

Your birth was a constricting band
denying you familiar dark circulation;
then a rush of air, gush of light
splashed you through the net of your mother,

slippery into your own body
into your own nine lives
and into the amateur hands
of your parent midwives:

One hand attached to a phone,
one holding a do-it-yourself book,
a third adjusting the bed and a fourth
basketting your pulsing head.

Born in a caul, coughed out of the belly
of the whale, wide-eyed, quivery.
Now blossoming into family flesh.
I wish you well in your human livery.

WATTLE-EYES

For JT, DB and TM

Like three Victorian explorers
camouflaged in khaki,
you stalked the drizzle,
black umbrellas overhead, binoculars poised,
while I trailed myopically behind
displaying a slouching, unfit jizz.

I faked, calling out like you
wet whisperings, lip trillings.
But it was no use, I did not see
the wattle-eyed flycatcher in the tangled bush
that after two hours showed its apparently
luminous, tiny, shy eye.

This gift you gave yourselves,
some other century's disciplined delight,
was a rebuke to shuffling me,
to my wattle-eyed and hooded sight.

TEXT OF NECESSITY

One by one
the small refusals
add up to a life.

Each returning home
is a scanter triumph.

You give and gain
scrupulous care, scrupulous blame,
won and lost and then reclaimed

to wear like polished bone:
an amulet to ward off and to hold

the present and the past,
their vacancies and weight,
and early outlines in white light.

What you want
becomes a set of words,
mirrors in your mouth.

Transpose this into necessity,
or make it plain

when you stifle, as you rename
the stirring of some
unscheduled love or pain.

NIGHT SPACE

The woman takes up all the space.
She spreads her legs
across the bed
as if she owns the place.

The man on the edge
of the occupied bed
can't decide if he wants
her sleeping perfume

or the neat-sheeted tomb
of a bed in a room
shuttered, uncluttered,
monadic, immune,

where all's effaced:
the woman's legs,
her careless spread,
her loose-limbed night embrace.

INNER NOTE

Like a wishbone
or the instep of your foot

this parabolic love curves,
wings stirring

in the neck nerves of a crane
at marsh's edge,

or bends its back into a kite
arching the membrane of blue flight

You breathe me out
I breathe you in

the smell of your skin
is salt and tide and tin.

The half-open door
tilts cooler light

upon the floor
and outside sounds come in,

an olive thrush
through the hibiscus bush

last evening note
throating me under you.

This much is all we have:
shadows gathering,

fugitive grace,
and the deep body as our penumbral space.

BRUSH STROKE

In the night a dream creases
you against me momentarily,
unfolding origami bird
in suspended rain, on a bending tree.

You brush beside me, the caress
guinea-fowl feathering my back.
Your dreaming leaves a ladder
leaning against a house of thatch.

You turn half in, half out of sleep
to lipread my dark silent mouth.
In our waking's slow ascent
I am the dream's aftertaste, its scent.

AUBADE

When I wake
and you have already
left the bed
(I hear you swirling
water in your mouth,
plugging the kettle in,
opening the side door
to the mountain),
I steal your pillow
for a moment, the plump one
your Yorkshire aunt
packed with duck feathers
in 1961, and I lay my head
on your head's imprint,
while downstairs your head fills up
with morning enterprise,
inventories, rehearsals, plans,
the day's new rustling feathers.

STAY HERE

For TM

Stay here, a little longer.
Stay here with me.

How easy it is for you to go,
step by step, print by print
as if you are just fetching
the washing off the line,
or stopping for the shopping
on your way from work,
just posting a subscription
for another year.

But ending up on another coast
where your dead are visiting overnight,
especially your wild friend
who wants your company so badly
he lies through his teeth,
promises if you stay night long,
there'll be wine, tobacco, debate,
and no women to call you back

importunately like this:
stay here a little longer, with me.

Poems from
Terrestrial Things

(2002)

SPRING CUSTOM

As is the custom,
all winter long the wild canary
in its cage inside the cellar
is fed and cared for.
It sings its buoyant song
as if still skybound,
till its notes quaver
and it sings no more
in the damp dark;
not even when the farmer
opens the wooden shutters
for a dose of daily cellular light.

Months later, before dawn,
an early stamp of boots
brings the man to his silent bird.
He lifts the cage, cloth still on top,
and walks towards the woods.
Shafts of moving light
and soil smells strong as coffee
slowly filter through the bars,
till, hooked high in a spreading chestnut
the uncovered cage sways like a lantern
among the buds and shoots
and blue sky feathering trees.

The bird hiccups, tests its unpadlocked voice,
and again, and then soars into song—
calling, we imagine, its lungs to free its wings.
And calling, as was planned, the new-born
and migrating birds of spring
to closer and exposed view.

In the chestnut, pert and curious,
a bird party sings
without shadow or memory,
perhaps exhorting the canary
to find a mate, or explain its habitat;
while it sings back
a duet we project our longings into,
despite our forebodings
because: there, we say,
are the trees, spring, and the wild birds
and there, the caged one about to be freed
and the farmer sharing the sun beside it.

But the farmer lifts his gun
and shoots as many as he can,
their bodies mostly too small to eat
though large enough
to spasm in the sky
before they fall
and are collected in a bag

on this bright morning
when now we hear
other guns shooting other birds
across the glittering Tuscan hills.

The caged canary,
shocked rigid
by the sudden shots,
smelling its betrayal
in gunpowder,
stops singing
until the following spring.

BIRDS AT BELLAGIO

Except for the undertaker-crows
sneering in sartorial black and gray
from elegant branches overhead,
the birds at Bellagio, small and large,
expect to die from gunshot wounds
on autumn afternoons.
So when Tony lifts his binoculars,
they shy from him as from a hunter,
into impenetrable green gloom,
their pewter throats sealing song
in the trussed cypresses that guard
mass graveyards of Italian birds,
shot once for food, and then for sport
through the venal centuries, in peace and war.

LIZARDS AT SAN MICHELE

At San Michele one anticipates
an underworld of coffin creatures:
eels oiling the island's undertow;
snakes camouflaged in leafy death mould
or sunning like long pastries on marble slabs;
bats poised on chapel cornices,
cartoon creations for the salons of the dead;
and faded chiffon moths
sucking from rosettes and wreaths.

But instead within the terracotta walls
it's all good cheer:
visitors with trowels and watering cans;
Ezra Pound, unexpectedly sensible
in his final domestic arrangements;
Brodsky, no longer coughing;
Diaghilev's stage-set adorned with ballet shoes;
and the fervent hospitality of waiter lizards,
electric servants of the dead.

MERCHANTS IN VENICE

We arrive in Venice to ancient acoustics:
the swaddling of paddle in water,
thud of the vaporetto against the landing site,
and the turbulent frescoes of corridors and ceilings,
belief and power sounding history
with the bells of the subdivided hour,
on water, air and all surfaces of light.

What have we Africans to do with this?
With holy water, floating graves and cypresses,
the adamantine intricacy of marble floors,
gold borders of faith, Mary's illuminated face
and the way Tintoretto's Crucifixion is weighted
with the burden of everyday sin and sweat,
while the city keeps selling its history and glass.

On the Rialto, tourists eye the wares
of three of our continent's diasporic sons,
young men in dreadlocks and caps, touting
leather bags and laser toys in the subdued dialect
of those whose papers never are correct,
homeboys now in crowded high-rise rooms
edging the embroidered city.

How did they get from Dakar to Venice?
What brotherhood sent them to barter and pray?
And on long rainy days when the basilica
levitates, dreaming of drowning,
do they think of their mission and mothers,
or hover and hustle like apprentice angels
over the shrouded campos and spires?

Into the city we have come for centuries,
buyers, sellers, mercenaries, spies,
artists, saints, the banished,
and boys like these: fast on their feet,
carrying sacks of counterfeit goods,
shining in saturated light,
the mobile inheritors of any renaissance.

PARTS OF SPEECH

Some stories don't want to be told.
They walk away, carrying their suitcases
held together with grey string.
Look at their disappearing curved spines.
Hunch-backs. Harmed ones. Hold-alls.

Some stories refuse to be danced or mimed,
drop their scuffed canes
and clattering tap-shoes,
erase their traces in nursery rhymes
or ancient games like blind man's buff.

And at this stained place words
are scraped from resinous tongues,
wrung like washing, hung on the lines
of courtroom and confessional,
transposed into the dialect of record.

Why still believe stories can rise
with wings, on currents, as silver flares,
levitate unweighted by stones,
begin in pain and move towards grace,
aerating history with recovered breath?

Why still imagine whole words, whole worlds:
the flame splutter of consonants,
deep sea-anemone vowels,
birth-cable syntax, rhymes that start in the heart,
and verbs, verbs that move mountains?

THE ARCHBISHOP CHAIRS THE FIRST SESSION

The Truth and Reconciliation Commission.
April 1996. East London, South Africa

On the first day
after a few hours of testimony
the Archbishop wept.
He put his grey head
on the long table
of papers and protocols
and he wept.

The national
and international cameramen
filmed his weeping,
his misted glasses,
his sobbing shoulders,
the call for a recess.

It doesn't matter what you thought
of the Archbishop before or after,
of the settlement, the commission,
or what the anthropologists flying in
from less studied crimes and sorrows
said about the discourse,
or how many doctorates,
books, and installations followed,
or even if you think this poem
simplifies, lionizes
romanticizes, mystifies.

There was a long table, starched purple vestment
and after a few hours of testimony,
the Archbishop, chair of the commission,
laid down his head, and wept.

That's how it began.

HOW TO MOURN IN A ROOM FULL
OF QUESTIONS

The witness tells it steady:
the breathing of a boy deep asleep
the way the young, even the watchful young, sleep;
the window splintering,
shaking shack walls,
raked breathing of the shot, same, boy.
The mother and her spreading blanket.

Old sorrow holds down anger like a plug.
And juridical questions
swab swab the brains and blood off the floor.

TONGUE-TIED

"Do you promise to tell the truth,
the whole truth and nothing but the truth?"

Someone's been hurt.
But she can't speak.
They say she's "tongue-tied".

Like an umbilical neck throttle.
No spit, sound, swallow.
Voice in a bottle.

Now she's speaking underwater,
to herself, to drowning,
to her son, her lost daughter.

Her tongue's a current
washing over dead fish,
abandoned rope and tackle:

"They came for the children, took, then me,
and then, then afterwards
the bucket bled. My ears went still.
I'm older than my mother when . . ."

The gull drags its wing to the lighthouse steps.
"That's the truth. So help. Whole. To tell."

WHAT KIND OF MAN?

TONY YENGENI: *"What kind of man are you? . . . I am talking about the man behind the wet bag."*
CAPTAIN JEFFREY T. BENZIEN: *". . . I ask myself the same question."*

—Cape Town Amnesty Hearings

I

It's the question we come back to.
After the political explanations
and the filmy flicker of gulags, concentration,
re-education and ethnic cleansing camps,
prisons and killings in the townships and fields,
here at the commission we ask again,
can't get away from it, leave it alone:
"What kind of man are you?"

II

What kind of man mounts another
in deadly erotic mimicry,
then puts a wet bag over his head
to suffocate him for "the truth"?

Lets her baby cry for her
from a nearby cell,
threatens to stop the crying?

Roasts meat on coals
while a man is burning on a nearby pyre?

Gives evidence like this
in daylight; but can give no account?

III

What kind of man are you?
What type? We ask and he asks too
like Victorians at a seminar.
Is it in the script, the shape of the head,
the family gene?
Graphology, phrenology or the devil?

IV

Nothing left but to screen his body.
We have no other measure
but body as lie detector,
truth serum, weathervane.

V

We look at his misshapen cheek,
how it turns away from questioning,
as if he's an abused child;

at his mouth, its elastic pantomime;

at his sagging chin, glottal Adam's apple,
throat no longer crisp from a morning razor;

at his eyes' pouches, pitted olives, dunes;

at the eyes themselves,
how they sweat, don't weep;

his ears, peaks on a listening uniform;

the hand with its thumb intact, its active fingers;

and the apparently depressed, possibly sedated,
shuffling lumbering cumbersome body
which then helpfully and earnestly
performs in slow motion with perfect memory
its training, its function: a tantric posture with wet bag
that just for a moment is so unbelievable
it looks like a pillow fight between brothers.

VI

Though of the heart we cannot speak
encased in its grille of gristle

the body almost but doesn't explain
"What kind of man are you?"

VII

This kind, we will possibly answer,
(pointing straight, sideways,
upwards, down, inside out):
this kind.

REVENGE OF THE IMAGINATION

"I would like to apologize before God . . . if ever I was to be employed,
I was going to poison the white man's children. The way they killed
my son hitting him against a rock . . . I will never forgive . . . I will
never rest . . . I used to go out and sleep on top of his grave."
—Ms Margaret Madlana, at Alexandra Township
Human Rights Violations testimony.

Margaret Madlana in the nursery of her imagination,
before God stays her mind, her hand,
puts rat poison in the ribena of the four-year-old
and in the schoolboy's warm breakfast milk:
and who can judge her?

Killing them in her heart
not so much to have them dead
(for they can never be as dead as her last born,
his broken head beside a murderous rock),
but that their parents might mourn for ever,
leaving the compact suburbs
each night for an expanding cemetery,
to lie upon the graves as she did,
unresting, unforgiving.

But there at the mounds' damp feet
they might also conjure in the dark
some symmetry for comfort,
an eye for an eye, a tooth for a tooth,
an eye and a tooth to body natural law.

Round and round and round we go
and which is the name of the next
in our broken circle
to be harmed for reckoning's sake—
the chosen one to briefly close
the metal ring, the open mouth of pain?

Tinker tailor soldier sailor
rich man poor man beggarman thief?

Which one, like Isaac,
his head on a rocky altar,
will we sacrifice in mind
to our dazed and shadowy
reverie of revenge, of recovery?

A COMMANDER GRIEVES ON HIS OWN

*"... If, in my professional language of expressing my regret that loved ones
have been lost and injured, if that is not sufficient, I apologize for that,
but that is how I feel. I am a soldier, and I have been taught to hide
my tears, and I have been taught to grieve on my own. ..."*
—Major General Marius Oelschig, head of the Ciskei Defence Force
at the time of the "Bisho Massacre".

You can't stop me hearing in the metre,
in this rhetoric of restraint,
the cadence of the vanquished.
Can't stop me thinking about defeated Roman generals
never profiled on busts and coins,
refused a culture's currency of honour.

We know bodies fell in disarray,
the wounded dragged across tangled lines,
false heroes jostling on all sides.
Fence blades shattered into shrapnel
and ignominious orders shouted
into blood and brokenness.

Asked to bear shame instead of arms,
to disclose motive and memory
in a confessional booth, a commander
in the court martial of his own judgement
must forgo public forgiveness,
hold mute his grief and guilt.

And I believe it may cost courage
to express professional decorums,
refuse the commerce of pardon
offered for a tale told with feeling,
waive absolution
in the forum of extracted truth.

I like to think instead
he opened his ruled heart in silence,
unpinned the old brazen medals
in a solitary corridor,
in solitary ceremony.

THE TRANSCRIBER SPEAKS

I was the commission's own captive,
Its anonymous after-hours scribe,
Professional blank slate.
Word by word by word
From winding tape to hieroglyphic key,
From sign to sign, I listened and wrote.
Like bricks for a kiln or tiles for a roof
Or the sweeping of leaves into piles for burning:
I don't know which:
Word upon word upon word.
At first unpunctuated
Apart from quotations and full stops.
But how to transcribe silence from tape?
Is weeping a pause or a word?
What written sign for a strangled throat?
And a witness pointing? That I described,
When officials identified direction and name.
But what if she stared?
And if the silence seemed to stretch
Past the police guard, into the street
Away to a door or a grave or a child,
Was it my job to conclude:
"The witness was silent. There was nothing left to say"?

THE SOUND ENGINEER

Of all the professionals engaged in Truth Commission reporting, the highest turn-over was apparently among reporters editing sound for radio.

From the speaker's mouth
through the engineer's ear,
sound waves of drought and flood
are edited for us to hear:
dunes filtering burnt desert sand,
corrupted wells, and shocks, shouts,
no longer muffled in the cochlea shell.

Listen, cut; comma, cut;
stammer, cut;
edit, pain; connect, pain; broadcast, pain;
listen, cut; comma, cut.
Bind grammar to horror,
blood heating the earphones,
beating the airwaves' wings.

For truth's sound bite,
tape the teeth, mouth, jaw,
put hesitation in, take it out:
maybe the breath too.
Take away the lips.
Even the tongue.
Leave just sound's throat.

Keep your ear to the ground,
to pain's surfacing,
its gulps for air, its low ragged flight
over history's topography.
The instrumental ear
records the lesions of eroded land
while blood drums the vellum of the brain.

A stain hovers like a small red butterfly
over the studio recording table
where the wall is listening,
so the ear dares to rest.
Then nothing.
Nothing but static,
insects invading air.

The sound engineer hears
his own tympanic membrane tear.

SOME THERE BE

"There be of them, that have left a name behind them, that their praises might be reported. And some there be, which have no memorial, who are perished as though they had never been; and are become as though they had never been born; and their children after them."
—Apocrypha

Only the rustle of reeds
thin pipe smoke
a flickering paraffin lamp
women in blankets bent over
their faces lost to the light.

And remnants:
gate without hinges
stones in a half circle
afterbirths buried in silt.

Can the forgotten
be born again
into a land of names?

BODY PARTS

may the wrist turn in the wind like a wing
the severed foot tread home ground

the punctured ear hear the thrum of sunbirds
the molten eye see stars in the dark

the faltering lungs quicken windmills
the maimed hand scatter seeds and grain

the heart flood underground springs
pound maize, recognize named cattle

and may the unfixable broken bone
loosened from its hinges

now lying like a wishbone in the veld
pitted by pointillist ants

give us new bearings.

STICKS ON STONE

I

What to remember returning home?
Use the prodding iron,

herd memories into a pen
especially the fattened one,

the thin one,
the one with the bent back leg

and the one we gave a name to,
the pretty one, the pretty one.

II

I am ten.
In a corner of the garden
the wind blows all day
through bluegum trees.
And see, here I am all grown up.

III

Absence makes the heart grow fonder,
the mind more furtive.

IV

Gather it all together at once
in an instant, into the grip of one hand:
people, places, shapes, weather, times,
then drop like pick-up sticks on stone,
observe intersections, scry the mirror
of the forgotten, read the bones.

V

Pure song: what's that?
Why do we hear a dying fall?

A FEW QUESTIONS

One died in utero, fully formed.
The other twin had wasted limbs
but became a real lady, dark-eyed,
fastidious, family cartographer
of birthdays, deathdays, feasts.

My mother, neighbours said,
had "her hands full" with the rest:
meaning my brother, her first
little fist to unfurl, then me,
spinning my hula hoop in a protective arc,
and the youngest girl,
who would take no help from anyone.

My father worked by day and by night.
When he "did sums" we whispered and watched.
The soles of our feet were country-hard.
Sun hit the stoep like a torpedo,
but no one slept in the hot afternoons
when tiny scorpions bred in a concrete basin
beside the servant's room.

Where was the dead baby buried?
Did Sputnik see us playing in the veld?
Couldn't Jesus make the lame to walk?
Would a sinkhole swallow our house and car?
If we had been quieter would the sums have added up?

FRIGHTENED OF THE DARK

For Kenneth at fifty

Your fear, at four, of the dark
is a family tale we hear again.

You're "sensitive", always were.
I've got "common sense", at two.
I'm walking down the airless passage to your room,
holding your hand, pulling up a chair,
climbing on it, switching on the light,
then checking under the bed to show you
there is no more dark, the dark is dead.

Both frightened of the dark,
of being crippled,
of our father who did art in heaven,
of rough boys on the street,
of sinkholes, of sounds outside,
of mother being unhappy.

But we had a pact, a deal,
humouring the fears, giving them shape.
One was scared, the other brave,
so that next time the roles could swop.

Long ago I climbed that chair,
my first chance to manage fright,
pretend that all was well
to get us through the southern night.

And now it's middle-age. You're in the north
where dark comes early,
seals the foreign cold.
Your turn to switch the light.

IN THE CAGE

Once a year I went underground,
to see what dad did, and to be brave.
After dressing up—hard hat angling a torch,
yellow overalls, oversized boots—the wait for the cage.
"Not the lift at John Orrs" my father's fellows joked
as it rattled up like a snake. Then the descent

into darkness, where flares torched us into the wet sinus
of the labyrinth and its precious artificial air,
to wires and cables crackling messages from the surface
and the ear-blistering hard judder of the jackhammers
cracking the centre of the earth,
where, as we children knew, miners would one day find
a bubbling volcano, China, or all the gold in the world.

The men below smiled shyly—
my mother said they missed their children—
but I was glad not to be the child
of an underground man,
eyes bloodshot, eardrums blown,
rattling in a cage, crawling through a cave,
while up above, only a curtain and a bed
and hot thick paste with gravy for food.

Orpheus and Eurydice confused me later:
somebody leaving, then turning back to look,
and somebody else going into the shuddering darkness.

SIRENS SOUNDING

When the familiar siren sounded
its high castrato peal,
some men surfaced, faces powdery,
sweat runnels down their arms,
and the shift boss barked
for the next ration of men
to take a last breath of cool air
and enter the tunnels again.

But then a longer wail,
keening Armageddon, everything at risk.
Nobody breathed till the count was in.
Even the children fell silent,
imagining the huddle of quietened men
at the staring headgear,
stretchers waiting with folded arms,
strained talk later at dinner.

WILLIAM KAMANGA

Today William Kamanga died,
he whom I loved and who maybe loved me.
A last picture eight months old:
wife and daughter holding a man
crumpled on a bench after a stroke.

William Kamanga served at our table
for thirty years before he retired.
Then each month my mother sent money and news.
Colonial circuits of care and demand,
love to hire and then to lose?

Short men with hands behind their backs
make me think of him.
Silvo and Nugget smell of his apron,
thousands of spoons and shoes polished
outside the kitchen in afternoon sun.

The Star, read quickly
on his bed raised on bricks,
refolded quickly before my father's return,
reminds me of his wary routine
when I crumple the daily news.

And Sunday afternoons, when visitors
who knew the dogs by name
sat outside in suits and ties,
talking softly about Banda
and the cost of transport home.

His pass, always trouble with Klerksdorp officials,
Mary, whom we hid from the black marias,
and his children, named twice,
once for themselves and once for us,
now lost to the city, dead of AIDS, working the fields.

Last year I went to Chinteche
having no fathers or uncles left,
no old man to show the way,
to discover him gone, a day's walk in the hills,
defending his rice from baboons and birds.

My phone messages hadn't reached him,
telegrams advising arrival hadn't come
and no one knew what to do with my sorrow.
Three grandchildren stood shyly in the shade
while in the kitchen Mary served tea

in my gran's teacups, on my sister's cross-stitch cloth,
while other familiars—Rhodesian copper vase,
ball-and-claw chair, old calendars on the dresser—
watched over us like Jesus and the ancestors.
And weeping for everything that had and hadn't happened,

we opened an album of photographs—
on one page William's high-domed head, paterfamilias,
on the next my mother's seventieth birthday smile
rearing like a sunflower in a field of cassava,
home from home.

MY FATHER'S BOOKS

My father's books move with me.
Across the Atlantic and back,
from mountain to sea views,
from storerooms to display.
Kept together, as a collection.
Kept for my mother, who hasn't the space,
for my siblings, for reference,
for old time's and sorrow's sake.

I never read my father's books.
Addison and Steele. John Stuart Mill.
Longfellow. Lamb's *Tales of Shakespeare*.
Thinkers, Everyman's, The Modern Library,
and records of two wars: his and the Boers'.
"Great Men" (Napoleon, Smuts, Lawrence of Arabia).
Leather school prizes, Brenthurst limiteds,
Streets of Johannesburg.

His autodidact's archive stores
grave truths I can't access.
Volumes stand firm, spines turn on me.
But I take care of them,
keep them behind glass,
their positions as stable as under his own gaze,
when they ordered his hardwon learning
like a neat, pragmatic wife.

I read instead his log books,
navigational codes I cannot understand,
aerodromes I cannot pronounce,
sorties, dusk raids, bombings,
to direct me up from the cased bindings
into the sky, his earlier, freer life.

A DEATH FORETOLD

Here to see you
say goodbye
rest my cheek
upon your hair.

Leaving you
I cross the road alone
holding my own hand.

Lights in three colours
send me forward, caution me
stop me in my tracks

as worlds wheel by
inside cars
where other mothers
turn their shining heads

towards some other
breathing child.

IN A NORTHERN CITY, SUDDENLY

Thought I recognized the tilt of his shoulder,
hands in both coat pockets,
and the cleft of his chin as he turned
blankly towards my radial gaze.

This happens to older travellers,
footsteps muted in foreign towns
where natives tread their stable streets
while strangers trace resemblances.

There are people visiting the Karoo
who claim it's just like Montana,
and in southern Ontario
find Transvaal shrubs and rocks.

And here in New York, seeing my father
wearing his old greatcoat,
head down, preoccupied as usual,
I wondered what he was up to.

But it wasn't him, couldn't have been.
This isn't the place, the time,
isn't even the hemisphere:
here I know no one's shoulder.

And he's meant to be dead,
not in northern time and space,
turning up here alone,
avoiding my glance again.

INTO THE SUN

This is where landscape comes to die.
Where the forlorn wind
wails a little, sags a little,
brooding in the bluegum trees
just as it used to.
Where Sunday afternoons
threaten weekdays
with fitful narcotic sleep.
Where by day the hot sun is flat
and by night the cold moon is flat,
petrified in the stretched horizon
that the eyes inspect
on their level journey home.

Two verticals: industry's acropolis,
the mine's meccano headgear,
crow's nest over empty compounds;
and abandoned mine dump middens,
gold's necropolis.

As before the only colour
other than ash and rock
is the sunset pyre, its bloody ink
dust motes beaten by disc ploughs,
a Tretchikoff painting glaring you down.

And inside the stooped
and stubborn silence
a few men still walk miles
along the main road
to somewhere else
much the same,
straight into the sun
without blinking.

THE HEAD OF THE HOUSEHOLD

is a girl of thirteen
and her children are many.

Left-overs, moulting gulls,
wet unweaned sacks

she carries them under her arms
and on her back

though some must walk beside her
bearing their own bones and mash

when not on the floor
in sickness and distress

rolled up in rows
facing the open stall.

Moon and bone-cold stars
navigational spoor

for ambulance, hearse,
the delivery vans

that will fetch and dispatch
the homeless, motherless

unclean and dead
and a girl of thirteen,

children in her arms,
house balanced on her head.

WOMEN AND CHILDREN FIRST

It's always been so.
This makes it worse.
Women and children first.

First to be hurt
last to be nursed.
It's always been so.

When rumour stalks
first to be cursed.
And worse.

Turned out, inside out.
Only safe in the hearse.
Women and children first.

THE CHILD AT THE LIGHTS

The child in the street
motions, asks for something.
Noon, a school day.
The car windows are steamy
but unopened to his mouthed request.
We have been told to keep doors locked fast.
We have been told to turn from
clamorous hands, tear ducts, miming necks.

All remember the call
for a hardened heart,
for welded arteries,
a wary pulse,
when children irrupt
at the traffic lights
at the threshold of the city.

For two hundred orphans
will soon be there, waiting for red.
In a long line their needs already sway.
Their satchels are packed with
two thousand brothers and sisters.
Two million more are in the wings.

COMPASSIONATE LEAVE

Almost everyone's on leave,
gone away

to the countryside,
in threadbare trucks

to pay respects
in rooms and huts

to watch and pray for dying ones
shrunken under sheets,

to vigils through the night
in closed-off streets

where grandmothers prepare
small and smaller funeral feasts

after truncated prayers
chanted by tired priests

over cardboard caskets
in the deathwatch heat.

Gone to taxi ranks and stations
to wait for information

from billboards, radios,
word of mouth and trumpets in the sky

where ubiquitous hadedas,
unlike Auden's mute impervious birds

blast their high shofars
over each infected space.

Body Maps

new poems

REPARATION

The action of restoring something to a proper or former state; spiritual restoration; the action of making amends for a wrong or loss; compensation for war damage by a defeated state.

What it cost no one is telling.
Can't subtract what might have been.
Can't add up to a sum we understand.
Can't subdivide what once was seen.

Can carve a tombstone for the dead,
memorialize with flowers and crosses,
exhume a body, clear a name,
issue receipts for wrongs and losses.

But can't repair, and can't restore
an uncut arm, unbruised genital,
untroubled sleep, unscarred face,
unweeping mother, children, faith
or wide unwatching private space.

TOO LONG A SACRIFICE

Too long a sacrifice
Can make a stone of the heart.
                    —Easter 1916, WB Yeats

The emptied shell
hears the pleated sea
grant clemency
to wrecks and submarines.

Forensic men
in the archive of modernity
interpret the statistics,
tell us things are getting better.

In boom times the suture holds.
The hungry share their begging bowls.
Demolished shacks rise from the dust.
"Life goes on." We're told it does.

But few who have been badly hurt
are ever healed. In the wounded heart
there lives a need to hurt in turn,
perhaps even to be hurt again.

For those who queue in cold dawn air,
uncounted by the census,
the hope barometer falls,
memory returns like weather.

Like drought and flood.
Lichen on a rock.
Like a rip tide
shuttling the unburied dead.

What to do? Watch and pray?
No benign conclusion waits
in the wings, enters to pull the curtain
down over hunger, grief and hate.

BRING THE STATUES BACK

Nobody lives in Verwoerdburg or Triomf anymore.
Names have changed,
some chiseled leaders of the past
now relocated or sold to foreigners.

Remember the gasp, the sheer delight:
(in memory filmed in black and white)
apartheid's architect a dangling man
at the end of a winch on a crane?

We hear he then was moved
to a garage in Bloemfontein
where his chipped statue friends
gaze at him disconsolately.

How easy, after all
to remove a world,
to erase a crooked line
and start again.

But the memory of a belted policeman,
his moustache like a dog on a leash—
let's not lose that, or we'll begin to believe
DRC church spires were darning needles.

And let's not forget suburban gates, dogs barking,
the duplicity of post office and liquor store.
If we auction the statue's buttons
we might forget the monumental overcoat.

Let's put Verwoerd back
on a public corner like a blister on the lips;
let's walk past him and his moulded hat,
direct traffic through his legs,
and the legs of his cronies of steel and stone.

IN TIMES OF WAR

The frog prince
dons a gas mask.

His breeding pond
is choked with smoke.

Migrating birds
can't find their way back.

Nobody's kissing
not even the air.

Statues lose breath,
suffer vertigo.

A thimble is a helmet
on a pointing finger.

Snares in the desert
corrugate the dunes.

Ploughshares turn
into tanks,

filigree to
rubble.

Veiled mourners
scatter ash confetti

in an out of season
carnevale.

And the dancing bear
only has one paw.

PILGRIMAGE

Take a trip, take a tour.
Go to newly bombed cities
to see what remains in the rubble,
scorched fragments or things saved whole.
Statues, courtyards, a wash of painting,
piazzas where people burned or still stroll,
mosaics, reliquaries in crypts,
holy sites, libraries, illuminated scrolls.

Visit Baghdad to scan what's left
of the beginnings of civilization,
Bamiyan to reassemble in your mind
giant sandstone Buddhas
from whose empty cocoons
flew the butterflies of the spirit.
See Madrid where Goya still accuses,
view the flattened towers of New York City,
ravaged Mogadishu and Beirut.

Then if you have time make a backward journey
to ancient Byzantium and Alexandria.
Traverse Bushman deserts and Aztec mounds
where memories hum in the sun.
Closer and closer, while some still remember the detail,
travel to Coventry, Warsaw, Dresden,
Hamburg and Hiroshima,
place your feet in the prints of the dead.

And then fast forward with your guide book
to cities undestroyed.
Go now. To still breathing
places of accumulated love and power,
where the line of a drawing,
an angle of light on a building,
a word's gravid pressure on a page
the sound of a ribbed instrument,
things made by hand, remade by eye or ear,
have not yet been forgotten, razed.

TREASURY

Meditation on the 2004 exhibition Curiosity CLXXV
at the University of Cape Town.

When we label and display
we entrust our traces to the past,
award them the prize of the present
or bequeath them
to a yet-to-be-discovered place.

In the cabinet of juxtaposed matter
each name, date and time
claims the space around itself,
reshapes it as a stage
for pageants or soliloquies.

Each object of discovery
sits like a mannequin,
a favoured child
beside competing siblings,
composed, mannerly, elbows in:
sarcoptes scabiei,
lead bars, ballet shoes,
platana frog,
waterproof field guide,
titanium implant, anteater.

Collection, exhibit, parade,
explication of signs.
These are our cables
to a signal box of meanings
underground or in the air.

Even if we believe
in other magic: divine purpose
and the syntax of the spirit
(some realm where
that-which-is mimics
that-which-will-be),
we are obliged to chronicle
in custodian grammar
the processes and particles of the earth,
to measure shape and weight,
retrieve history,
reach into the future.

Talisman, relic, fetish, portent:
we rub up against them like cats.

The resurrection plant,
its drought resistant gene.
A bird's blood temperature,
demography, flight politics.
Seasonal calendar revealed
by dassies' tiny teeth.
The heart in foreign lodging.
Lost language, fugitive tracks,
their tracings on paper or in paint.

In graph, key, index we profess
that what we make and remake
in our laboratories of meaning
compasses the sphere
of nature and generation.

But the world holds up
its torn arm, torn wing,
an angel or horseman
reining us in, as we enter
the archive of half-known things
with our quiver of blunt arrows.

"THE FEAR OF GOD IS THE BEGINNING OF KNOWLEDGE"

—Billboard. Liwaladzi Village, Malawi

Out there where knowledge begins
on the outskirts of a village,
prayers are chanted at the side of the road,
women swirl round and round
with their eyes turned in
and the priest from the nearby town
collecting a few kwachas for the mission
preaches today about tongues,
teaches how they descended like
fiery crows onto the fields.
Then some possessed by the gift of fire
begin speaking in tongues
and others say nothing
and the fear of God is at hand.

Out there where God begins
we see and read the billboard on the sandy road
and are warned as we drive past in sin,
as we drive past talking and eating,
reading a guidebook with our radio on
and pointing at the hungry tongues,
which lap like commas in the sky.

BODY MAPS

For Harriette Yeckel

Take the body   trace its outline
map its armature
tendons   viscera   scar tissue
fractures   swellings
promises and wishes.
Map age   genes   place of origin
and love's lineaments.

For mapped onto each body is love.

Cartography of one's own country
or the contours of a foreign land.

A journey through forests
over cataracts
turbulent rivers   peaks
ravines   rift valleys
grasslands   wetlands
oceans   sand.
Down mine shafts.
Through truck stops.
In towns and cities.
On tarred roads   dirt tracks.

At the shoreline is a flare
where pain's fire
consumes itself
with its earth-hunger
unquenched thirst
burning wings.

It lights the way
back to touch
soft or violent
stretched or shortened
above   below
where there are sounds
soft calls   moans
fright   resistance   silence
movements
towards or away
where there is rupture or seeping
where openings are buds
that shrink or blossom
where the spine buckles
or uncurls
where nails draw blood
or declawed fingers
touch tip to tip
and palms dance.

Mapped onto each body is
that first launch into love:
parachute drop of our begetters
and then each body's own
open or closed arms and legs.

And onto the bodies of those
who die of love's lesions
we map our love too
guilty shadow tracings
lucky escape routes
provisional survival.

Take your own body
or the leached body
of your mother   your father
your brother   your sister.
Transparent body
of glass   of leaves
of encoded messages
to the past and the future
unique thumbprint maze
ubiquitous death mask.

Take it trace it map it remember.

THRENODY

Thin waxen boys and girls
Sunken eyes, shrunken gaze
Ashen hearts and rusted veins
All to come to dust.

So lively once
Your eyes ablaze.
With lungs of crimson
Lungs robust

You sang the street, the sun.
The earth turned round and round.
On rare clear nights we shared with you
The moon's crisp golden crust.

Now we face your stares
Children stacked in tombs.
Your glazed eyes pursue us
Through the catacombs.

We yearn to reconnect your bones
Hold up your necks and heads;
Our hope to rise with you
In the first coup of the dead.

WISHING IN MOONLIGHT

For the "hunchback" man at Camphill Village

The midnight moon alights on his back,
hitches a ride to heaven.
His hunch is a cresset-light,
Dick Whittington, a circus tent
a call to alms, a sack of dreams.
It's a conch, cosmic backpack,
the ocean's echo as the tide turns.

Not laden, not burdened,
he's buoyed by the light of the moon.
The helium balloon on his vertebral vine
lifts him off the grit on the ground
where roots and dongas
threaten his stumbling walk,
raises him up up up,
above the dark alleys that corner him,
the creophagous cathedral that lies,
above false rumours and shame,
above the straightbacks and their stares,
turned-down mouths and unbending spines.

Helium, lightest of the noble gases,
drug of the gods and of those flying solo
carries him over the surgery,
its masks and scalpels,
above the pain of the ever-bent
and floats him into a blue-domed room
where salve is served on silver platters
and his lungs fill at last to the brim,
where everyone crooked is beaming
and everyone's mother is there.

CHILD STRETCHING

—After Santu Mofokeng's photograph "Vaalrand Farm"

This is not my child.
This is not my child's stretching shadow.
Not my enamel basin,
wedding ring, torn dress,
not me bending to wash
the breakfast plates, the boy on his toes
or the other small torso who waits a turn
for water or attention.

I think this is the boy who may grow tall
—he is already practising—
who will stride through Africa
—look at his sturdy legs—
this Vaalrand boy with his joyful stretch.
Never mind the cold morning.
Never mind the colder water.
Never mind the corrugated curtain.

This is not my child.
Nor is his assiduous mother my friend.
But her loving proximity
makes me, here just outside the frame,
(I know, you don't have to tell me,
in the simplest, most suspect way),
makes me want to be her sister,
her child my buoyant nephew.

LETTER FROM CHILDHOOD

We're told that a childhood of scars
is assured. Whether your mother's face

was a star, a mask, deflated like a balloon
or mirrored your own fixed face:

scars, scars. And not just mothers.
Someone or something terrible turns you

into a victim or killer; some in-between thing
suspends your breath at night, chokes you in the morning;

some not-so-bad but not exactly great thing
makes you a loner, poet, stutterer.

Why then the letter posted long ago
arriving at dawn on the wind
with its old sweet news?

The sheets on the washing line
billow like angels, not shrouds.

After running home, dry breath
plumes horse tails in cold scrub air.

Mother and father are spied
kissing in the garden, even if only once.

Friends hold hands at school;
tenderness breaks out everywhere.

A crippled sister wobbles, walks.
A brother's infectious laugh

as he reads *Just William*
by torchlight a room away

creases a household as
smiles zig zag down the hall.

We all knew the veld
could raise its angry fur

but a seasonal fire
we could, we did, put out.

WHEN CHILDREN LEAVE

They have to go: all children need to leave,
give up their childish things. Open the champagne!
It's no use hoping for a last reprieve.

We're in this century, we're not naïve.
The bags are packed, down comes the rain.
They need to go: all children have to leave

to show they're grown: that's what we believe.
Though in some cultures children do remain
at home, don't hope so for a last reprieve.

It wouldn't help to self-deceive,
to think they would be happier here. It's plain
they need to go, all children have to leave.

It's not as if we plan to weep and cleave
to them. Pick up their bags, walk firmly to the train.
It's no use hoping for a last reprieve.

They'll visit us; their love can be retrieved
if we can feign good cheer, our poise retain.
They have to go: all children need to leave.
It's no use hoping for a last reprieve.

WILL

To her son, only child,
her collection of frames
and three gold rings
from a graveyard of loves.
Two Kruger rands.
Six cool throats of cut crystal.
Her "death in service" benefits.
Recently edited,
an album of photographs
of other dead people
and well known landmarks
around the world.
His early drawings,
letters, birthday cards.
A file labelled "destroy
before reading"
which he will probably read.
As is her way
nothing forgotten,
everything willed.

NOTES FOR THAT WEEK

—After Seferis

❦

Friday

The sun throws its net
of peremptory shadows.
Across the road
noisy renovations,
then removal of rubble.

The doctor says the graph
is a source for concern.
He doesn't know
your arrhythmic heart
is playing a jazz theme.

Saturday

Remember, inaugural day
nineteen ninety-four,
our table piled with the future?
From the window we watched
three men in the street
search our garbage bin
for bread or bottles,
liberation's left-overs.

Sunday

I never get lost in the city streets
because I follow the same route,
park in the same lot,
visit the same bookshop
eat outdoors
have a cell phone ready.

There are some changes:
a building implodes,
on the foreshore a new one
aspires to interpret the century.
Men from the Congo
their eyes border-crossing,
safeguard the cars
in courteous French.
There are more children
though some are taller,
grow older, as we do.

Monday

On the corner a man
sells mobiles of yachts, cheap string

fraying in the hot wind.
His dog hardly stirs; nobody buys.

Tuesday

Women who live alone are precise.
In the laboratory of feeling
a pantry, preserves arranged
according to colour, date, size.
Kumquat, green fig, apricots in brandy.

Wednesday

The south-easter blows.
Wednesday's child is full of woe.

Thursday

Inside.
The house with the cool rooms in summer.
High ceilings, white mouldings.
Light filters through wooden blinds
onto books, sharpened pencils,
an unpolished desk, a silent telephone.
Who is sleeping away the long afternoon?

Outside.
The washing line shrouded by sheets
in the concrete courtyard.
Green mosaic of mint, sage and beans
and cheap red jewels: tomatoes, zagreb chillies.
The lime tree and its lightbulbs.
Frangipani dropping
unseasonal yellow and white tears
onto unmown grass.
The nuzzle of the sea breeze
in the greying fur of the cat.

DEATH ARRIVES

It never occurs the way one predicts
It never does.

It won't ever disclose the year or hour
It only contradicts.

No matter which way you are facing
No notice is given, no notice taken.

It seldom erupts like a corner brawl
Or a TV countdown to space or war.

It may arrive with a message or none at all
With a mouth stitched up, or a babe in a caul.

It may be a hangman, or dangling noose
It may or may not play fast, play loose.

Could have an aim or have no such thing
Could hang its intent on its arm like a sling.

It hurries alone, or slowly is led
By a ring in its nose, with a wreath on its head

To the office, the courtyard,
House, road or bed

Whichever path leads
To the broken dead

Round and round
Up and down
To the broken dead.

DEATH NOTICES

Death notices
in column inches.
Alphabetizes, capitalizes.
"Always Remembered"
"Bravely Suffered, Bravely Borne"
"Cremation at 4 pm"
"Private Ceremony"
"Donations in lieu of flowers"

Then it notices
how many people
attend the wake
write a letter
place an ad
send flowers
how many care to phone in
and after a month a year
it notices again
who still remembers
the recent dead

Death notices
the stammer of the priest
the scuffling of feet
the choice of hymns
quavering at the high notes
Rock of ages, cleft for me
or predictable Psalm 23

Death notices
it notices you
in your old grey suit
waiting in the queue
to the open casket
you kneeling
for the first time in years
age marks
upon your hands
you afterwards reeling
in the bright sun

TIME TO GO

For Antjie Krog and John Samuel

It's time to go.
We've been at the door
For some time.
The other guests
Left long ago
Trailing their scarves
Like excuses behind them.
But here we are again
Always the last to go
Carrying trays
Of liquor glasses
To the kitchen
Catching a last stray
Word or joke
Then talking at the car
With the doors open
For another half hour.
I want dying to be like this.
A lingering lazy farewell
After dinner and conversation
Till the host thinks: "Enough!
It's 2 am. These people have to go."

THE ECLIPSE OF THE SUN

Limpopo Province, 4 December 2002

I

In December the sun
was eclipsed by the moon.

A wind swept from behind our backs,
cast beating wings, a shadow pall,

a cold grey coat over us,
then kidnapped breath.

Earth's hearth went silent and dark.
Silent and dark and cold.

Call it neutral. Or cruel.
Or scriptural.

Hair quills hardened on hands and necks.

For eighty-four seconds
we watched for the sign

that darkness would pass,
our bones keep their heat,

the earth not turn
to fossil and stone.

II

And then just on time the sun a poached egg
rose from its steaming pan

almost predictable again,
a crinoline of rays flared back,

a chariot trailing clouds,
an angel of God ascending.

III

Some watchers cheered,
some threw up their arms, some bent their heads.

In the light our irises normalized,
we could see each other,

subdued, but wearing familiar expressions,
helping young and old to their feet.

Larks winged back from night
into day, over grass and seed

and then soft rain began to fall,
as they had said it might.

KALAHARI CAMPSITE

In the Kalahari night we wonder at stars—
above us so far, so many, all indelible—
we think we're underneath them, they're in space and time
beyond us, we're small and fleshy and they are adamantine

but then immediately it's raining stars, it's shooting stars
the whole world is stars and nothing else
desert dunes, red sand, wild cats on killing raids
brown-backed hyena at the fire's burnt remains
an owl's alarm call, the pattern of ants across stone
they're all stars, and we too are stars
we glitter, we rotate, we fall away
we are nothing, there is nothing, but stars

Sketches from a Summer Notebook

new poems

LETTER HOME

From me in an Umbrian castle to you at home

Light sieves through cheesecloth,
thickens overnight into morning fog,
then dense air turns to blue.

By noon sunflowers are twisting their necks
to follow the sun, and when it's gone,
they will twist back again.

It's as if in the desert a cactus waves its handless arms
at our passing car, we think "Tequila ad"
and don't wave back, driving on.

But I have no driver's license
and you are far away raking leaves
pruning, pulling out weeds.

Your views are mountain, sea, and sky
but perhaps today on the verandah
the wind blows rain into your eyes.

Wasps refuse to fly out of my windows
though there is nothing sweet in here.
I am too scared to chase them away
so hide in a shuttered room.

When I am not hiding from wasps
the view from my windows is this:
a lane of cypresses, stone houses,
an elegant polygamous white rooster,

lucerne, those sunflowers,
and mealies in papyrus sheaves
that make me cheer though
I have never grown a mealie patch and hate putu.

The geraniums in the terracotta pots
around the castle are ours, damn it.
Mine. I want our pelargoniums and clivia back,
and the plumbago too if they don't mind.

Please come soon! To eat gelato, see the sights,
(twenty-six species still sing)
protect me from the wasps' mean sting
and foreign thefts or slights.

UMBRIAN SHUTTERS

They open at five to public light.
Outside life mows and clears the hills.
They open to farmers, tractors,
crows and golden fields.
They open to hay bales rolled tight
tilting as if to cartwheel
down the highway to Rome.
They signal to a white wisp of cloud
soon to be scorched burnt blue.

At two o'clock the shutters close
and inside smudges centuries.
The house shuts its face to the street,
rebuffs requests, says: "No!
I have a private life. I have a blind eye too."
And the dark that settles on the bed,
cupboard and other heavy furniture
dusts them of light,
lets everything die for the afternoon.

WALKING BACK LATE AT NIGHT

Inside an aisle of cypresses
my torch makes shadows of shadows,
darting fireflies darn the dark,
gravel crackles underfoot,
and now I pass the chicken shed
where beaks and throats are quiet inside
resting till morning's crow.

How can I walk so lightly in this dark?
Where a body pressed against a tree
could menace me by watching
or a blade could jag across my path
and pierce my heart or brain tonight.

But no, I am safe in this dark,
I am blessed, I am lucky,
only the weight of honeysuckle is upon me,
tall indifferent trees around me,
only fireflies glance and glitter,
nothing is watching me, nothing.

SOLITAIRE AT FRONZOLA

For Jonathan Cohen

In the chapel room a small window
open to the summer air
decants vintage light over my sheet.
My eyes are bright as fever.
Everyone else is curtained, and asleep.

No wolves, no prayers, no torture rack.
Only the moon, it's angled light,
deconsecrated shadows,
and my torso carrara marble
mottled white.

LA TRAVIATA

Violetta spun, a cocoon
Unravelling, a ribbon
Unfurling on a kite.
When after three hours
She sang her last note, sank and died
In her white ruffled nightdress
On the outdoor stage in rural Umbria
We were all amazed
And applauded like rock star fans.
But I want her checked for bruises
Now that she is alive again
And on a bus to the next town
With Alfredo, the travelling Latvian orchestra
And the rest of the crew.

SUNFLOWERS

In case you think
the sunflowers in the field
are always on summer holiday,
florid fools raising
oil-stained cheeks
like drunks in a bar,
you are wrong.

Believe me:
that yellow and the deep furry eye
is Apollo's camouflage, aka God.
They're allies of the sun,
timepieces on the landscape's wrist
and van Gogh and Blake are visiting this afternoon
to tell us what they mean
and how we too should grow and live.

IN THE CHIMNEY

In the chimney—sweet bird song!
No bird falls down stunned
into the empty grate
or bearing grass in its beak
makes a purgatorial base
half-way between fire and sky.
Just a chimney sweeper's chorus
cleaning winter's smoke with song.

About the Author

Ingrid de Kok has published three previous collections of poetry, *Familiar Ground*, *Transfer* and *Terrestrial Things*. *Seasonal Fires* is her first book to be published in the United States. She lives in South Africa.